FRONTOTEMPORAL DISORDERS

Information for Patients, Families, and Caregivers

LEARN ABOUT:
- Frontotemporal dementia
- Primary progressive aphasia
- Movement disorders

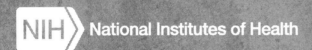 National Institutes of Health

National Institute on Aging
National Institute of Neurological Disorders and Stroke

The National Institute on Aging (NIA) and the National Institute of Neurological Disorders and Stroke (NINDS) are part of the National Institutes of Health, the nation's medical research agency—supporting scientific studies that turn discovery into health.

NIA leads the federal government effort conducting and supporting research on aging and the health and well-being of older people. NIA's Alzheimer's Disease Education and Referral (ADEAR) Center offers information and publications on dementia and caregiving for families, caregivers, and professionals.

NINDS is the nation's leading funder of research on the brain and nervous system. The NINDS mission is to reduce the burden of neurological disease.

For additional copies of this publication or further information, contact:

National Institute on Aging
Alzheimer's Disease Education and Referral Center
www.nia.nih.gov/alzheimers
1-800-438-4380

National Institute of Neurological Disorders and Stroke
www.ninds.nih.gov
1-800-352-9424

CONTENTS

Introduction

Few people have heard of frontotemporal disorders, which lead to dementias that affect personality, behavior, language, and movement. These disorders are little known outside the circles of researchers, clinicians, patients, and caregivers who study and live with them. Although frontotemporal disorders remain puzzling in many ways, researchers are finding new clues that will help them solve this medical mystery and better understand other common dementias.

The symptoms of frontotemporal disorders gradually rob people of basic abilities—thinking, talking, walking, and socializing—that most of us take for granted. They often strike people in the prime of life, when they are working and raising families. Families suffer, too, as they struggle to cope with the person's daily needs as well as changes in relationships and responsibilities.

This booklet is meant to help people with frontotemporal disorders, their families, and caregivers learn more about these conditions and resources for coping. It explains what is known about the different types of disorders and how they are diagnosed. Most importantly, it describes how to treat and manage these difficult conditions, with practical advice for caregivers. A list of resources begins on page 27.

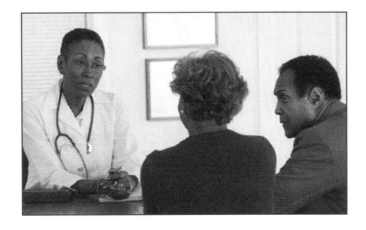

The Basics of Frontotemporal Disorders

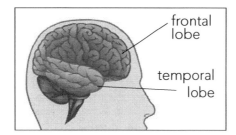

frontal lobe

temporal lobe

Frontotemporal disorders are the result of damage to neurons (nerve cells) in parts of the brain called the frontal and temporal lobes. As neurons die in the frontal and temporal regions, these lobes atrophy, or shrink. Gradually, this damage causes difficulties in thinking and behaviors normally controlled by these parts of the brain. Many possible symptoms can result, including unusual behaviors, emotional problems, trouble communicating, difficulty with work, or difficulty with walking.

A Form of Dementia

Frontotemporal disorders are forms of dementia caused by a family of brain diseases known as frontotemporal lobar degeneration (FTLD). Dementia is a severe loss of thinking abilities that interferes with a person's ability to perform daily activities such as working, driving, and preparing meals. Other brain diseases that can cause dementia include Alzheimer's disease and multiple strokes. Scientists estimate that FTLD may cause up to 10 percent of all cases of dementia and may be about as common as Alzheimer's among people younger than age 65. Roughly 60 percent of people with FTLD are 45 to 64 years old.

People can live with frontotemporal disorders for up to 10 years, sometimes longer, but it is difficult to predict the time course for an individual patient. The disorders are progressive, meaning symptoms get worse over time. In the early stages, people may have just one type of symptom. As the disease progresses, other types of symptoms appear as more parts of the brain are affected.

No cure or treatments that slow or stop the progression of frontotemporal disorders are available today. However, research is improving awareness and understanding of these challenging conditions. This progress is opening doors to better diagnosis, improved care, and, eventually, new treatments.

FTD? FTLD? Understanding Terms

One of the challenges shared by patients, families, clinicians, and researchers is confusion about how to classify and label frontotemporal disorders. A diagnosis by one doctor may be called something else by a second, and the same condition or syndrome referred to by another name by a pathologist who examines the brain after death.

For many years, scientists and physicians used the term *frontotemporal dementia* (FTD) to describe this group of illnesses. After further research, FTD is now understood to be just one of several possible variations and is more precisely called *behavioral variant frontotemporal dementia*, or bvFTD.

This booklet uses the term *frontotemporal disorders* to refer to changes in behavior and thinking that are caused by underlying brain diseases collectively called *frontotemporal lobar degeneration* (FTLD). FTLD is not a single brain disease but rather a family of neurodegenerative diseases, any one of which can cause a frontotemporal disorder (see "Causes," page 11). Frontotemporal disorders are diagnosed by physicians and psychologists based on a person's symptoms and results of brain scans and genetic tests. With the exception of known genetic causes, the type of FTLD can be identified definitively only by brain autopsy after death.

Changes in the Brain

Frontotemporal disorders affect the frontal and temporal lobes of the brain. They can begin in the frontal lobe, the temporal lobe, or both. Initially, frontotemporal disorders leave other brain regions untouched, including those that control short-term memory.

The frontal lobes, situated above the eyes and behind the forehead both on the right and left sides of the brain, direct executive functioning. This includes planning and sequencing (thinking through which steps come first, second, third, and so on), prioritizing (doing more important activities first and less important activities last), multitasking (shifting from one activity to another as needed), and monitoring and correcting errors.

What's going on?

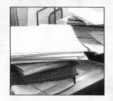

Brian, an attorney, began having trouble organizing his cases. In time, his law firm assigned him to do paperwork only. Brian's wife thought he was depressed because his father had died 2 years earlier. Brian, 56, was treated for depression, but his symptoms got worse. He became more disorganized and began making sexual comments to his wife's female friends. Even more unsettling, he neither understood nor cared that his behavior disturbed his family and friends. As time went on, Brian had trouble paying bills and was less affectionate toward his wife and young son. Three years after Brian's symptoms began, his counselor recommended a neurological evaluation. Brian was diagnosed with bvFTD.

When functioning well, the frontal lobes also help manage emotional responses. They enable people to avoid inappropriate social behaviors, such as shouting loudly in a library or at a funeral. They help people make decisions that make sense for a given situation. When the frontal lobes are damaged, people may focus on insignificant details and ignore important aspects of a situation or engage in purposeless activities. The frontal lobes are also involved in language, particularly linking words to form sentences, and in motor functions, such as moving the arms, legs, and mouth.

The temporal lobes, located below and to the side of each frontal lobe on the right and left sides of the brain, contain essential areas for memory but also play a major role in language and emotions. They help people understand words, speak, read, write, and connect words with their meanings. They allow people to recognize objects and to relate appropriate emotions to objects and events. When the temporal lobes are dysfunctional, people may have difficulty recognizing emotions and responding appropriately to them.

Which lobe—and part of the lobe—is affected first determines which symptoms appear first. For example, if the disease starts in the part of the frontal lobe responsible for decision-making, then the first symptom might be trouble managing finances. If it begins in the part of the temporal lobe that connects emotions to objects, then the first symptom might be an inability to recognize potentially dangerous objects—a person might reach for a snake or plunge a hand into boiling water, for example.

Types of Frontotemporal Disorders

Frontotemporal disorders can be grouped into three types, defined by the earliest symptoms physicians identify when they examine patients.

- **Progressive behavior/personality decline**—characterized by changes in personality, behavior, emotions, and judgment (called behavioral variant frontotemporal dementia).

- **Progressive language decline**—marked by early changes in language ability, including speaking, understanding, reading, and writing (called primary progressive aphasia).

- **Progressive motor decline**—characterized by various difficulties with physical movement, including the use of one or more limbs, shaking, difficulty walking, frequent falls, and poor coordination (called corticobasal syndrome, supranuclear palsy, or amyotrophic lateral sclerosis).

In the early stages it can be hard to know which of these disorders a person has because symptoms and the order in which they appear can vary widely from one person to the next. Also, the same symptoms can appear later in different disorders. For example, language problems are most typical of primary progressive aphasia but can also appear later in the course of behavioral variant frontotemporal dementia. The table on page 6 summarizes the three types of frontotemporal disorders and lists the various terms that could be used when clinicians diagnose these disorders.

Trouble with words

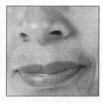

Alicia's first symptom was trouble talking. She spoke more slowly and thought she sounded stilted. She could under-stand people well enough, but finding the right words when she was talking became harder and harder. Also, Alicia, 49, could not write words like "and" and "it" but could write words like "alligator." Her doctor recommended a neurological exam, which helped diagnose agrammatic PPA.

Types of Frontotemporal Disorders

Diagnostic Terms	Main Early Symptoms
Progressive Behavior/Personality Decline	
• Behavioral variant frontotemporal dementia (bvFTD) • Temporal/frontal variant FTD (tvFTD, fvFTD) • Pick's disease	• Apathy, reduced initiative • Inappropriate and impulsive behaviors • Emotional flatness or excessive emotions • Memory generally intact
Progressive Language Decline	
• Primary progressive aphasia (PPA) • Progressive nonfluent aphasia • Semantic dementia	• Semantic PPA (also called semantic dementia): can't understand words or recognize familiar people and objects • Agrammatic PPA (also called progressive nonfluent aphasia): omits words that link nouns and verbs (such as to, from, the) • Logopenic PPA: trouble finding the right words while speaking, hesitation, and/or pauses in speech
Progressive Motor Decline	
• Corticobasal syndrome (CBS)	• Muscle rigidity • Difficulty closing buttons, operating simple appliances; difficulty swallowing • Language or spatial orientation problems
• Progressive supranuclear palsy (PSP)	• Progressive problems with balance and walking • Slow movement, falling, body stiffness • Restricted eye movements
• FTD with parkinsonism	• Movement problems similar to Parkinson's disease, such as slowed movement and stiffness • Changes in behavior or language
• FTD with amyotrophic lateral sclerosis (FTD-ALS)	• Combination of FTD and ALS (Lou Gehrig's disease) • Changes in behavior and/or language • Muscle weakness and loss, fine jerks, wiggling in muscles

Behavioral Variant Frontotemporal Dementia

The most common frontotemporal disorder, *behavioral variant frontotemporal dementia* (bvFTD), involves changes in personality, behavior, and judgment. People with this dementia can act strangely around other people, resulting in embarrassing social situations. Often, they don't know or care that their behavior is unusual and don't show any consideration for the feelings of others. Over time, language and/or movement problems may occur, and the person needs more care and supervision.

In the past, bvFTD was called Pick's disease, named after Arnold Pick, the German scientist who first described it in 1892. The term Pick's disease is now used to describe abnormal collections in the brain of the protein tau, called "Pick bodies." Some patients with bvFTD have Pick bodies in the brain, and some do not.

Primary Progressive Aphasia

Primary progressive aphasia (PPA) involves changes in the ability to communicate—to use language to speak, read, write, and understand what others are saying. Problems with memory, reasoning, and judgment are not apparent at first but can develop over time. In addition, some people with

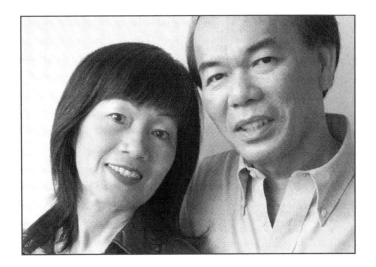

"What do you mean by salt?"

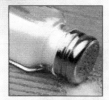

Jane, 62, a university professor, began having trouble remembering the names of common objects while she lectured. She also had a hard time following conversations, especially when more than one person was involved. Her family and co-workers were unaware of Jane's difficulties—until she had a hard time recognizing longtime colleagues. One night at the dinner table, when Jane's husband asked her to pass the salt, she said, "Salt? What do you mean by salt?" He took her to a neurologist, who diagnosed semantic PPA. As her illness progressed, Jane developed behavioral symptoms and had to retire early.

PPA may experience significant behavioral changes, similar to those seen in bvFTD, as the disease progresses.

There are three types of PPA, categorized by the kind of language problems seen at first. Researchers do not fully understand the biological basis of the different types of PPA. But they hope one day to link specific language problems with the abnormalities in the brain that cause them.

In *semantic PPA*, also called semantic dementia, a person slowly loses the ability to understand single words and sometimes to recognize the faces of familiar people and common objects.

In *agrammatic PPA*, also called progressive nonfluent aphasia, a person has more and more trouble producing speech. Eventually, the person may no longer be able to speak at all. He or she may eventually develop movement symptoms similar to those seen in corticobasal syndrome.

In *logopenic PPA*, a person has trouble finding the right words during conversation but can understand words and sentences. The person does not have problems with grammar.

Movement Disorders

Two rare neurological disorders associated with FTLD, *corticobasal syndrome* (CBS) and *progressive supranuclear palsy* (PSP), occur when the parts of the brain that control movement are affected. The disorders may affect thinking and language abilities, too.

CBS can be caused by corticobasal degeneration—gradual atrophy and loss of nerve cells in specific parts of the brain. This degeneration causes progressive loss of the ability to control movement, typically beginning around age 60. The most prominent symptom may be the inability to use the hands or arms to perform a movement despite normal strength (called apraxia). Symptoms may appear first on one side of the body, but eventually both sides are affected. Occasionally, a person with CBS first has language problems or trouble orienting objects in space and later develops movement symptoms.

PSP causes problems with balance and walking. People with the disorder typically move slowly, experience unexplained falls, lose facial expression, and have body stiffness, especially in the neck and upper body—symptoms similar to those of Parkinson's disease. A hallmark sign of PSP is trouble with eye movements, particularly looking down. These symptoms may give the face a fixed stare. Behavior problems can also develop.

Other movement-related frontotemporal disorders include *frontotemporal dementia with parkinsonism* and *frontotemporal dementia with amyotrophic lateral sclerosis* (FTD-ALS).

Confusing symptoms

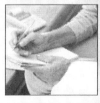

Carol had a tingling sensation and numbness in her upper right arm. Then her arm became stiff. She had to change from cursive handwriting to printing. Carol, 61, told her doctor that she had trouble getting her thoughts out and described her speech as "stumbling." She had increasing trouble talking but could still understand others. Eventually, she was diagnosed with CBS.

Trouble with walking

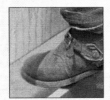 For a year and a half, John had trouble walking and fell several times. He also had trouble concentrating. He couldn't read because the words merged together on the page. John, 73, also seemed less interested in social activities and projects around the house. His wife noticed that he was more irritable than usual and sometimes said uncharacteristically inappropriate things. John's primary care doctor did several tests, then referred him to a neurologist, who noted abnormalities in his eye movements and diagnosed PSP.

Frontotemporal dementia with parkinsonism can be an inherited disease caused by a genetic tau mutation. Symptoms include movement problems similar to those of Parkinson's disease, such as slowed movement, stiffness, and balance problems, and changes in behavior or language.

FTD-ALS is a combination of bvFTD and ALS, commonly called Lou Gehrig's disease. Symptoms include the behavioral and/or language changes seen in bvFTD as well as the progressive muscle weakness seen in ALS. Symptoms of either disease may appear first, with other symptoms developing over time. Mutations in certain genes have been found in some patients with FTD-ALS.

Causes

Frontotemporal lobar degeneration (FTLD) is not a single brain disease but rather a family of brain diseases that share some common molecular features. Scientists are beginning to understand the biological and genetic basis for the changes observed in brain cells that lead to FTLD.

Scientists describe FTLD in terms of patterns of change in the brain seen in an autopsy after death. These changes include loss of neurons and abnormal amounts or forms of proteins called tau and TDP-43. These proteins occur naturally in the body and help cells function properly. When the proteins don't work properly and accumulate in cells, for reasons not yet fully understood, neurons in specific brain regions are damaged.

In most cases, the cause of a frontotemporal disorder is unknown. In about 15 to 40 percent of people, a genetic (hereditary) cause can be identified. Individuals with a family history of frontotemporal disorders are more likely to have a genetic form of the disease than those without such a history.

Familial and inherited forms of frontotemporal disorders are often related to mutations (permanent changes) in certain genes. Genes are basic units of heredity that tell cells how to make the proteins the body needs to function. Even small changes in a gene may produce an abnormal protein, which can lead to changes in the brain and, eventually, disease.

Scientists have discovered several different genes that, when mutated, can lead to frontotemporal disorders:

* **Tau gene (also called the MAPT gene)**—A mutation in this gene causes abnormalities in a protein called tau, which forms tangles inside neurons and ultimately leads to the destruction of brain cells. Inheriting a mutation in this gene means a person will almost surely develop a frontotemporal disorder, usually the bvFTD form, but the exact age of onset and symptoms cannot be predicted.

- **PGRN gene**—A mutation in this gene can lead to lower production of the protein progranulin, which in turn causes TDP-43, a cellular protein, to go awry in brain cells. Many frontotemporal disorders can result, though bvFTD is the most common. The PRGRN gene can cause different symptoms in different family members and cause the disease to begin at different ages.

- **VCP, CHMP2B, TARDBP, and FUS genes**—Mutations in these genes lead to very rare familial types of frontotemporal disorders. TARDBP and FUS gene mutations are more often associated with hereditary ALS.

- **C9ORF72 gene**—An unusual mutation in this gene appears to be the most common genetic abnormality in familial frontotemporal disorders and familial ALS. It also occurs in some cases of sporadic ALS. This mutation can cause a frontotemporal disorder, ALS, or both conditions in a person.

Scientists are continuing to study these genes and to search for other genes and proteins, as well as nongenetic risk factors, that may play a role in frontotemporal disorders. They are trying to understand, for example, how mutations in a single gene lead to different frontotemporal disorders in members of the same family. Environmental factors that may influence risk for developing the disorders are also being examined.

Families affected by inherited and familial forms of frontotemporal disorders can help scientists further research by participating in clinical studies and trials. For more information, talk with a health care professional, contact any of the research centers listed at the end of this booklet, or search *www.clinicaltrials.gov.*

Diagnosis

No single test, such as a blood test, can be used to diagnose a frontotemporal disorder. A definitive diagnosis can be confirmed only by a genetic test in familial cases or a brain autopsy after a person dies. To diagnose a probable frontotemporal disorder in a living person, a doctor—usually a neurologist, psychiatrist, or psychologist—will:

- record a person's symptoms, often with the help of family members or friends

- compile a personal and family medical history

- perform a physical exam and order blood tests to help rule out other similar conditions

- if appropriate, order testing to uncover genetic mutations

- conduct a neuropsychological evaluation to assess behavior, language, memory, and other cognitive functions

- use brain imaging to look for changes in the frontal and temporal lobes.

Different types of brain imaging may be used. A magnetic resonance imaging (MRI) scan shows changes in the size and shape of the brain, including the frontal and temporal lobes. It may reveal other potentially treatable causes of the person's symptoms, such as a stroke or tumor. In the early stage of disease, the MRI may appear normal. In this case, other types of imaging, such as positron emission tomography (PET) or single photon emission

Is it depression?

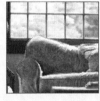

Ana's husband was the first to notice a change in his 55-year-old wife's personality. Normally active in her community, she became less interested in her volunteer activities. She wanted to stay home, did not initiate conversations, and went on her daily walks only if her husband suggested it. Ana's family thought she might be depressed. A psychologist recognized that her cognition was impaired and referred her to a neurologist, who diagnosed bvFTD.

Can't find the right words

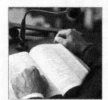

Ray, 60, was a small-town minister, a quiet intellectual, and a poet. He had always been thoughtful and well spoken, but over time his weekly sermons became halting and confused. He had trouble finding the right words and resorted to gestures. His family doctor thought that Ray had had a stroke. But when tests showed no stroke, she referred Ray to a university medical center, where specialists diagnosed logopenic PPA.

computed tomography (SPECT), may be useful. PET and SPECT scans measure activity in the brain by monitoring blood flow, glucose usage, and oxygen usage. Other PET scans can help rule out a diagnosis of Alzheimer's.

Frontotemporal disorders can be hard to diagnose because their symptoms—changes in personality and behavior and difficulties with speech and movement—are similar to those of other conditions. For example, bvFTD is sometimes misdiagnosed as a mood disorder, such as depression, or as a stroke, especially when there are speech or movement problems. To make matters more confusing, a person can have both a frontotemporal disorder and another type of dementia, such as Alzheimer's disease. Also, since these disorders are rare, physicians may be unfamiliar with the relevant symptoms and signs.

Getting the wrong diagnosis can be frustrating. Without knowing their true condition, people with frontotemporal disorders may not get appropriate treatment to manage their symptoms. Families may not get the help they need. People lose valuable time needed to plan treatment and future care. The medical centers listed on pages 29–30 of this booklet are places where people with frontotemporal disorders can be diagnosed and treated.

Researchers are studying ways to diagnose frontotemporal disorders earlier and more accurately. One area of research involves biomarkers, such as proteins or other substances in the blood or cerebrospinal fluid, which can be used to measure the progress of disease or the effects of treatment. Also being studied are ways to improve brain imaging, including seeing the tau protein, and neuropsychological testing, which assesses learning, language, problem solving, memory, and other thinking skills.

Common Symptoms

Symptoms of frontotemporal disorders vary from person to person and from one stage of the disease to the next as different parts of the frontal and temporal lobes are affected. In general, changes in the frontal lobe are associated with behavioral symptoms, while changes in the temporal lobe lead to language and emotional disorders.

Symptoms are often misunderstood. Family members and friends may think that a person is misbehaving, leading to anger and conflict. For example, a person with bvFTD may neglect personal hygiene or start shoplifting. It is important to understand that people with these disorders cannot control their behaviors and other symptoms. Moreover, they lack any awareness of their illness, making it difficult to get help.

Behavioral Symptoms

* **Problems with executive functioning**—Problems with planning and sequencing (thinking through which steps come first, second, third, and so on), prioritizing (doing more important activities first and less important activities last), multitasking (shifting from one activity to another as needed), and self-monitoring and correcting behavior.

* **Perseveration**—A tendency to repeat the same activity or to say the same word over and over, even when it no longer makes sense.

* **Social disinhibition**—Acting impulsively without considering how others perceive the behavior. For example, a person might hum at a business meeting or laugh at a funeral.

* **Compulsive eating**—Gorging on food, especially starchy foods like bread and cookies, or taking food from other people's plates.

* **Utilization behavior**—Difficulty resisting impulses to use or touch objects that one can see and reach. For example, a person picks up the telephone receiver while walking past it when the phone is not ringing and the person does not intend to place a call.

Language Symptoms

- **Aphasia**—A language disorder in which the ability to use or understand words is impaired but the physical ability to speak properly is normal.

- **Dysarthria**—A language disorder in which the physical ability to speak properly is impaired (e.g., slurring) but the message is normal.

People with PPA may have only problems using and understanding words or also problems with the physical ability to speak. People with both kinds of problems have trouble speaking and writing. They may become mute, or unable to speak. Language problems usually get worse, while other thinking and social skills may remain normal for longer before deteriorating.

Embarrassing behavior

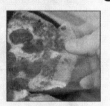 David and his wife ran a successful store until he began to act strangely. He intruded on his teenaged daughters' gatherings with friends, standing and staring at them but not realizing how embarrassed they were. He took food from other people's plates. A year later, David, 47, and his wife lost their business. After a misdiagnosis of depression and no improvement, David's wife took him to a neurologist, who diagnosed bvFTD.

Emotional Symptoms

- **Apathy**—A lack of interest, drive, or initiative. Apathy is often confused with depression, but people with apathy may not be sad. They often have trouble starting activities but can participate if others do the planning.

- **Emotional changes**—Emotions are flat, exaggerated, or improper. Emotions may seem completely disconnected from a situation or are expressed at the wrong times or in the wrong circumstances. For example, a person may laugh at sad news.

- **Social-interpersonal changes**—Difficulty "reading" social signals, such as facial expressions, and understanding personal relationships. People may lack empathy—the ability to understand how others are feeling—making them seem indifferent, uncaring, or selfish. For example, the person may show no emotional reaction to illnesses or accidents that occur to family members.

Not acting like himself

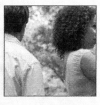

Previously a devoted husband, Gary began an extramarital affair at age 55—and didn't care that everyone knew about it. His wife was devastated and angry. His friends agreed that this was not like him. All attempts to reason with him were unsuccessful, as Gary could not understand how his actions hurt others. His wife insisted on a visit to the doctor. Initially, Gary was misdiagnosed with bipolar disorder. After further evaluation, he was told he had bvFTD.

Movement Symptoms

- **Dystonia**—Abnormal postures of body parts such as the hands or feet. A limb may be bent stiffly or not used when performing activities that are normally done with two hands.

- **Gait disorder**—Abnormalities in walking, such as walking with a shuffle, sometimes with frequent falls.

- **Tremor**—Shakiness, usually of the hands.

- **Clumsiness**—Dropping of small objects or difficulty manipulating small items like buttons or screws.

- **Apraxia**—Loss of ability to make common motions, such as combing one's hair or using a knife and fork, despite normal strength.

- **Neuromuscular weakness**—Severe weakness, cramps, and rippling movements in the muscles.

Treatment and Management

So far, there is no cure for frontotemporal disorders and no way to slow down or prevent them. However, there are ways to manage symptoms. A team of specialists—doctors, nurses, and speech, physical, and occupational therapists—familiar with these disorders can help guide treatment.

Managing Behavior

The behaviors of a person with bvFTD can upset and frustrate family members and other caregivers. It is natural to grieve for the "lost person," but it is also important to learn how to best live with the person he or she has become. Understanding changes in personality and behavior and knowing how to respond can reduce caregivers' frustration and help them cope with the challenges of caring for a person with a frontotemporal disorder.

Changing the schedule

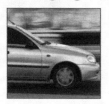

Matthew, 53, diagnosed with bvFTD, insisted on playing the card game solitaire on the computer for hours every morning. He did not care that this activity interfered with his wife's schedule. His wife figured out how to rearrange her day to stay home in the morning and take Matthew on errands and appointments in the afternoon. A portable device for solitaire in the car helped distract him.

Managing behavioral symptoms can involve several approaches. To ensure the safety of a person and his or her family, caregivers may have to take on new responsibilities or arrange care that was not needed before. For example, they may have to drive the person to appointments and errands, care for young children, or arrange for help at home.

It is helpful, though often difficult, to accept rather than challenge people with behavioral symptoms. Arguing or reasoning with them will not help because they cannot control their behaviors or even see that they are unusual or upsetting to others. Instead, be as sensitive as possible and understand that it's the illness "talking."

18

Frustrated caregivers can take a "timeout"—take deep breaths, count to 10, or leave the room for a few minutes.

To deal with apathy, limit choices and offer specific choices. Open-ended questions ("What would you like to do today?") are more difficult to answer than specific ones ("Do you want to go to the movies or the shopping center today?").

Maintaining the person's schedule and modifying the environment can also help. A regular schedule is less confusing and can help people sleep better. If compulsive eating is an issue, caregivers may have to supervise eating, limit food choices, lock food cabinets and the refrigerator, and distract the person with other activities. To deal with other compulsive behaviors, caregivers may have to change schedules or offer new activities.

Medications are available to treat certain behavioral symptoms. Antidepressants called selective serotonin reuptake inhibitors are commonly prescribed to treat social disinhibition and impulsive behavior. Patients with aggression or delusions sometimes take low doses of antipsychotic medications. The use of Alzheimer's disease medications to improve behavioral and cognitive symptoms in people with bvFTD and related disorders is being studied, though results so far have been mixed, with some medications making symptoms worse. If a particular medication is not working, a doctor may try another. Always consult a doctor before changing, adding, or stopping a drug.

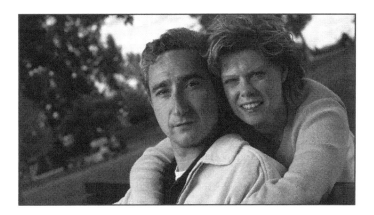

Treating Language Problems

Treatment of primary progressive aphasia (PPA) has two goals—maintaining language skills and using new tools and other ways to communicate. Treatment tailored to a person's specific language problem and stage of PPA generally works best. Since language ability declines over time, different strategies may be needed as the illness progresses.

To communicate without talking, a person with PPA may use a communication notebook (an album of photos labeled with names of people and objects), gestures, and drawings. Some people find it helpful to use or point to lists of words or phrases stored in a computer or personal digital assistant.

Finding a new way to communicate

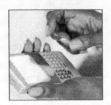 Mary Ann, a television news anchor for 20 years, began having trouble reading the nightly news. At first, her doctor thought she had a vision problem, but tests showed that her eyesight was normal. Although normally creative and energetic, Mary Ann, 52, had trouble finishing assignments and voicing her ideas at staff meetings. In time, she was let go from her job. Mary Ann applied for Social Security disability benefits, which required a medical exam. Her symptoms puzzled several doctors until a neurologist diagnosed logopenic PPA. A speech therapist taught Mary Ann to use a personal digital assistant to express words and phrases. For emergencies, Mary Ann carries a card in her wallet that explains her condition.

Caregivers can also learn new ways of talking to someone with PPA. For example, they can speak slowly and clearly, use simple sentences, wait for responses, and ask for clarification if they don't understand something.

A speech-language pathologist who knows about PPA can test a person's language skills and determine the best tools and strategies to use. Note that many speech-language pathologists are trained to treat aphasia caused by stroke, which requires different strategies from those used with PPA. (See the Resources section starting on page 27 to find speech-language pathologists and other experts who know about frontotemporal disorders.)

Managing Movement Problems

No treatment can slow down or stop frontotemporal-related movement disorders, though medications and physical and occupational therapy may provide modest relief.

For people with corticobasal syndrome (CBS), movement difficulties are sometimes treated with medications for Parkinson's disease. But these medicines offer only minimal or temporary improvement. Physical and occupational therapy may help people with CBS move more easily. Speech therapy may help them manage language symptoms.

For people with progressive supranuclear palsy (PSP), sometimes Parkinson's disease drugs provide temporary relief for slowness, stiffness, and balance problems. Exercises can keep the joints limber, and weighted walking aids—such as a walker with sandbags over the lower front rung—can help maintain balance. Speech, vision, and swallowing difficulties usually do not respond to any drug treatment. Antidepressants have shown modest success. For people with abnormal eye movements, bifocals or special glasses called prisms are sometimes prescribed.

People with FTD-ALS typically decline quickly over the course of 2 to 3 years. During this time, physical therapy can help treat muscle symptoms, and a walker or wheelchair may be useful. Speech therapy may help a person speak more clearly at first. Later on, other ways of communicating, such as a speech synthesizer, can be used. The ALS symptoms of the disorder ultimately make it impossible to stand, walk, eat, and breathe on one's own.

For any movement disorder caused by FTLD, a team of experts can help patients and their families address difficult medical and caregiving issues. Physicians, nurses, social workers, and physical, occupational, and speech therapists who are familiar with frontotemporal disorders can ensure that people with movement disorders get appropriate medical treatment and that their caregivers can help them live as well as possible.

The Future of Treatment

Researchers are continuing to explore the genetic and biological actions in the body that lead to frontotemporal disorders. In particular, they seek more information about genetic mutations that cause FTLD, as well as the disorders' natural history and disease pathways. They also want to develop better ways, such as specialized brain imaging, to track its progression, so that treatments, when they become available, can be directed to the right people. The ultimate goal is to identify possible new drugs and other treatments to test.

Researchers are also looking for better treatments for frontotemporal disorders. Possible therapies that target the abnormal proteins found in the brain are being tested in the laboratory and in animals. Clinical trials and studies are testing a number of possible treatments in humans.

Clinical trials for individuals with frontotemporal disorders will require many participants. People with frontotemporal disorders and healthy people may be able to take part. To find out more about clinical trials, talk to your health care provider or visit *www.clinicaltrials.gov*.

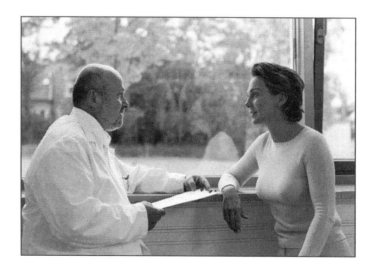

Caring for a Person with a Frontotemporal Disorder

In addition to managing the medical and day-to-day care of people with frontotemporal disorders, caregivers can face a host of other challenges. These challenges may include changing family relationships, loss of work, poor health, decisions about long-term care, and end-of-life concerns.

Family Issues

People with frontotemporal disorders and their families often must cope with changing relationships, especially as symptoms get worse. For example, the wife of a man with bvFTD not only becomes her husband's caregiver, but takes on household responsibilities he can no longer perform. Children may suffer the gradual "loss" of a parent at a critical time in their lives. The symptoms of bvFTD often embarrass family members and alienate friends. Life at home can become very stressful.

Changing relationships

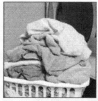

After Justin graduated from college, he went home to live with his parents for a short time. It didn't take long to notice personality changes in his 50-year-old mother, a successful executive. She became more childlike and had trouble finishing household chores. By the time she was diagnosed with bvFTD, Justin's relationship with his mother had deteriorated. Learning about the disorder helped Justin understand and accept the changes he was seeing in his mother.

Work Issues

Frontotemporal disorders disrupt basic work skills, such as organizing, planning, and following through on tasks. Activities that were easy before the illness began might take much longer or become impossible. People lose their jobs because they can no longer perform them. As a result, the caregiver might need to take a second job to make ends meet—or reduce hours or even quit work to provide care and run the household. An employment attorney can offer information and advice about employee benefits, family leave, and disability if needed.

Workers diagnosed with any frontotemporal disorder can qualify quickly for Social Security disability benefits through the "compassionate allowances" program. For more information, see *www.socialsecurity.gov/ compassionateallowances* or call 1-800-772-1213.

Caregiver Health and Support

Caring for someone with a frontotemporal disorder can be very hard, both physically and emotionally. To stay healthy, caregivers can do the following:

- Get regular health care.

- Ask family and friends for help with child care, errands, and other tasks.

- Spend time doing enjoyable activities, away from the demands of caregiving. Arrange for respite care—short-term caregiving services that give the regular caregiver a break—or take the person to an adult day care center, a safe, supervised environment for adults with dementia or other disabilities.

- Join a support group for caregivers of people with frontotemporal disorders. Such groups allow caregivers to learn coping strategies and share feelings with others in the same position.

The organizations listed in the Resources section of this booklet (starting on page 27) can help with information about caregiver services and support.

A stressful disorder

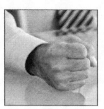 Robert, 60, started humming and whistling throughout the day. Over time, his humming got louder, and he started banging on the table over and over again. Robert's wife and his boss at work were concerned about this behavior and tried to distract him, but this became stressful for everyone. Robert lost his job. A doctor diagnosed bvFTD and prescribed medication to control his behavior. Robert began to attend an adult day services program.

Long-Term Care

For many caregivers, there comes a point when they can no longer take care of the person with a frontotemporal disorder without help. The caregiving demands are simply too great, perhaps requiring around-the-clock care. As the disease progresses, caregivers may want to get home health care services or look for a residential care facility, such as a group home, assisted living facility, or nursing home. The decision to move the person with a frontotemporal disorder to a care facility can be difficult, but it can also give caregivers peace of mind to know that the person is safe and getting good care. The decreased level of stress may also improve the caregivers' relationship with his or her loved one.

End-of-Life Concerns

People with frontotemporal disorders typically live 6 to 8 years with their conditions, sometimes longer, sometimes less. Most people die of problems related to advanced disease. For example, as movement skills decline, a person can have trouble swallowing, leading to aspiration pneumonia, in which food or fluid gets into the lungs and causes infection. People with balance problems may fall and seriously injure themselves.

It is difficult, but important, to plan for the end of life. Legal documents, such as a will, living will, and durable powers of attorney for health care and finances, should be created or updated as soon as possible after a diagnosis of bvFTD, PPA, or a related disorder. Early on, many people can understand and participate in legal decisions. But as their illness progresses, it becomes harder to make such decisions.

A physician who knows about frontotemporal disorders can help determine the person's mental capacity. An attorney who specializes in elder law, disabilities, or estate planning can provide legal advice, prepare documents, and make financial arrangements for the caregiving spouse or partner and dependent children. If necessary, the person's access to finances can be reduced or eliminated.

Conclusion

It is impossible to predict the exact course of frontotemporal disorders. These disorders are not easy to live with, but with help, people can meet the challenges and prepare for the future. Getting an early, accurate diagnosis and the right medical team are crucial first steps. Researchers and clinicians are working toward a deeper understanding of frontotemporal disorders and better diagnosis and treatment to help people manage these difficult conditions.

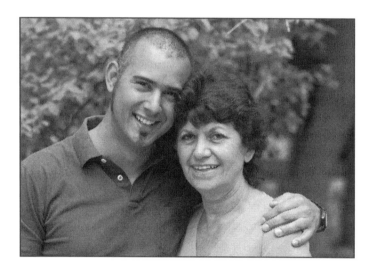

Resources

Federal Government

National Institute on Aging
Alzheimer's Disease Education and Referral (ADEAR) Center
P.O. Box 8250
Silver Spring, MD 20907-8250
1-800-438-4380 (toll-free)
www.nia.nih.gov/alzheimers

National Institute of Neurological Disorders and Stroke
P.O. Box 5801
Bethesda, MD 20894
1-800-352-9424 (toll-free)
www.ninds.nih.gov

MedlinePlus
National Library of Medicine
www.medlineplus.gov

Organizations

Association for Frontotemporal Degeneration
Radnor Station Building 2, Suite 320
290 King of Prussia Road
Radnor, PA 19087
1-267-514-7221
1-866-507-7222 (toll-free)
www.theaftd.org

ALS Association
27001 Agoura Road, Suite 250
Calabasas Hills, CA 91301-5104
1-800-782-4747 (toll-free)
www.alsa.org

CurePSP
30 East Padonia Road, Suite 201
Timonium, MD 21093
1-800-457-4777
www.curepsp.org

National Aphasia Association
350 Seventh Avenue, Suite 902
New York, NY 10001
1-800-922-4622 (toll-free)
www.aphasia.org

Caregiver Services

Eldercare Locator
1-800-677-1116 (toll-free)
www.eldercare.gov

Family Caregiver Alliance
785 Market Street, Suite 750
San Francisco, CA 94103
1-800-445-8106 (toll-free)
www.caregiver.org

National Academy of Elder Law Attorneys, Inc.
1577 Spring Hill Road, Suite 220
Vienna, VA 22182
1-703-942-5711
www.naela.org

Caregiver Support

Association for Frontotemporal Degeneration Support Groups
www.theaftd.org/support-resources/finding-support/caregiver-support-groups

FTD Support Forum
www.ftdsupportforum.com

PPA Support Group
www.groups.yahoo.com/group/PPA-support

Well Spouse Association
63 West Main Street, Suite H
Freehold, NJ 07728
1-800-838-0879
www.wellspouse.org

Diagnosis, Treatment, and Research Centers

Columbia-Presbyterian Medical Center
Lucy G. Moses Center for Memory and Behavioral Disorders
New York, NY
1-212-305-6939
http://cumc.columbia.edu/dept/neurology/memory

Indiana University School of Medicine
Indiana Alzheimer's Disease Center
Indianapolis, IN
1-317-278-5500
http://iadc.iupui.edu

Johns Hopkins University School of Medicine
Frontotemporal Dementia and Young-Onset Dementias Clinic
Baltimore, MD
1-410-502-2981
*www.hopkinsmedicine.org/Psychiatry/specialty_areas/neuropsychiatry/
frontotemporal_dementia*

Massachusetts General Hospital
Frontotemporal Disorders Unit
Boston, MA
1-617-726-5571
www.ftd-boston.org

Mayo Clinic
Department of Neurology
www.mayoclinic.org/frontotemporal-dementia

Rochester, MN
1-507-538-3270
www.mayoclinic.org/frontotemporal-dementia/rsttreatment.html

Jacksonville, FL
1-904-953-0853
www.mayoclinic.org/frontotemporal-dementia/jaxtreatment.html

Scottsdale, AZ
1-800-446-2279
www.mayoclinic.org/frontotemporal-dementia/scttreatment.html

Northwestern University Feinberg School of Medicine
Cognitive Neurology and Alzheimer's Disease Center
Chicago, IL
1-312-908-9339
www.brain.northwestern.edu

University of California, Los Angeles
Frontotemporal Dementia & Neurobehavior Clinic
Los Angeles, CA
1-310-794-2550
www.ftd.ucla.edu/clinic

University of California, San Francisco
Memory and Aging Center
San Francisco, CA
1-415-476-6880
www.memory.ucsf.edu/ftd

University of Pennsylvania Health System
Penn Frontotemporal Degeneration Center
Philadelphia, PA
1-215-349-5863
http://ftd.med.upenn.edu

Acknowledgments

NIH thanks the following people for their contributions to the vision and creation of this booklet:

Darby Morhardt, PhD, LCSW
Research Associate Professor
Director of Education, Cognitive Neurology and Alzheimer's Disease Center
Northwestern University Feinberg School of Medicine

Sandra Weintraub, PhD
Professor of Psychiatry and Behavioral Sciences
Clinical Core Leader, Cognitive Neurology and Alzheimer's Disease Center
Northwestern University Feinberg School of Medicine

Jennifer Merrilees, RN, MS
Clinical Nurse Specialist
Department of Neurology
Memory and Aging Center
University of California, San Francisco

Catherine Pace-Savitsky, MA
Former Executive Director
Association for Frontotemporal Degeneration

Susan Dickinson, MS, CGC
Executive Director
Association for Frontotemporal Degeneration

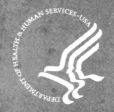

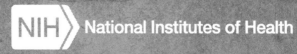

National Institutes of Health

Publication No. 14-6361
June 2014

33598256R00022

Made in the USA
Middletown, DE
16 January 2019